Under Cover Of Demons

BY

Geula Salomonova

A Memoir About

Paranoid Schizophrenia

Disorder

gsalomonova@gmail.com

All Rights Reserved © 2014

Table of Content

Introduction	4
Summoning a Devil	6
Marriage	11
Migrating to Israel	14
In Israel	17
Studying at the University	21
True Love	24
Meeting Yigal	25
Working as A Programmer	33
Meeting the Devil	43
Hospitalization at "Tower" Mental Hospital	53
Life After the Hospital	67
The Second Time in "Tower" Mental Hospital	81
Living in The USA	99

Trip to Las Vegas	101
Woman-Snake	103
The Third Stroke of Schizophrenia	105
Another Meeting with The Devil	111
Meeting Malcolm	116
Crazy Days	129
Wayne Dyer	141
In Canada	143
Back to Israel	145
Sanity	147

Introduction

This is the life story of Geula Salomonova. It is based on real life events. Geula is ill with the mental disorder called Paranoid Schizophrenia. The story is told from her point of view. This means that many events that are hallucinations might sound like fiction, but they are real. Nothing is fictional.

There are a lot of medical books and other materials on schizophrenia, but not much has been said from first hand experience. Those who are sick will never tell you their tale. This is because they are not coherent and not in touch with their surroundings most of the time. Thus their point of view and experience are kept secret. Geula, who passed through the usual psychotic experiences, had the good fortune of overcoming them and being able to tell her story. However, although the act of writing of this book was not easy, Geula decided to make the effort to finish it and share it with you.

The book can be seen as the memoirs of a woman who has been haunted by Satan and demons. The whole story takes place through various countries and from the age of 15 to 36. The names of the characters have been changed to protect their identity and privacy. From this point on I will narrate as Geula. Seven years have passed since the events of this story took place.

The inspiration for writing this book was from reading Anita Moorjani's *Dying to Be Me*. It narrates her life story and tells about a woman dying from cancer, but eventually coming back to life. Thus, I decided to tell you about what had happened in my life.

Summoning a Devil

I was born in 1974 on New Year's Eve. When I was a teenager, at the age of 15, I lived in a village in Bryansk district in Russia with my mother. My father was not living with us because my parents divorced when I was two years old.

Every evening the village youngsters gathered together to have fun. We used to get together in the village club, playing cards, listening to music and sometimes dancing. We used to hang around and drink vodka outside the club. Sometimes guys from neighboring villages came to our place. They came by riding horses, driving tractors or just walking.

One evening two men came over. One of them was named "Boss". This was his nickname. The other man's name I cannot recall. We sneaked into an abandoned house and sat down on the beds. Boss told me that his friend was crazy. I was eager to ask him what had happened with him. At that age I wanted to know everything. I came up to him and asked: "What bothers you? How did this happen?".

He replied: "You don't want to know. It's dangerous". But I insisted; I wanted to know it badly. I persuaded him, and he told me that he had tried to summon the Devil and one night he had seen somebody's hand crawling from beneath the bed. I asked him to teach me how to summon the Devil. He agreed to do it and started explaining, "Take a mirror and scissors, tie a thread to the scissors and spin it on the mirror's surface".

When I came back home I decided to try it. I tied a thread to the scissors and started spinning it on the mirror. I whispered that I wanted to become rich in exchange for my soul. But the Devil never came and nothing happened. I was just a young girl back then and had no idea what a terrible mistake I had made. I was to meet the Devil much later.

Some time later I was lying in my bed and heard somebody casting stones at my window. "It must be the guys",

I thought and looked out of the window. It was dark but I could discern a black figure in a black hat. He stood silent.

I asked him: "Who are you? What do you want?" He said nothing. He stood there for a while and then rushed to the bushy fence and disappeared.

Next morning, I examined the place where the Man in Black vanished. Not even a cat could fit through this narrow hole, but the Man in Black had disappeared without a trace.

I loved the city of Riga in Latvia where I was born. Some time later I visited Riga to see my friends and when I returned I was about to start culinary studies in the city Dmitrov. From Riga I brought some bubblegum that I was going to sell to my college friends. Back then, after the fall of communism, there was a lack of food and imported bubblegum was a luxury. I started selling the bubblegum: ten Rubles per pack. But no one wanted to buy. Everybody was just taking a bar and saying that they would give me the money for it later.

In the end no one paid. I got very mad and even attacked one girl, tearing off her necklace. Due to that incident I did not want to return to that college. I went back to the village in Bryansk for the weekend. When the time came to go back to the college, I got the on the train and suddenly changed my mind. I decided to go to Lvov in Ukraine instead, to try and apply for the horse taming college there. I had loved horses since childhood.

Once I boarded the train I realized that the passenger car was empty. I was alone. It was night time so I decided to go to sleep. In Russian trains you can sleep in the passenger car. As soon as I fell asleep there came a strange feeling of complete numbness. I could not move a muscle, could not wake up, and suddenly I felt some strange ray of light reaching me. Some flux was filling my head. I woke up finally and sat down on the couch. I looked through the window and saw a big star moving parallel to the train. There was no one but me in the wagon, and I was scared.

I arrived in Lvov, but I failed to get into the horse taming college, so I had to go home empty-handed. The whole trip took three days. When I got home, my mother was thrilled. She said she had called the police to search for me.

Marriage

When I was nineteen years old my mother and I moved to Yaroslavl, to my grandmother's place. I worked at a race track as a horse breaker. For all my life my mother tried to get rid of me. She tried to send me to an orphanage when I was a child. She and my grandmother tried to rent a room in order to get me off their backs; I was a drag for both of them.

One day my mother said to me in cold blood: "Go away". I got extremely mad at her, took my belongings, boarded the train and headed to Saint Petersburg to search for a better life. I rented an apartment and started my own business selling clothes at the market.

I met a man there. His name was Slava and he was selling jackets. We exchanged telephone numbers and soon he called me inviting me to his place. I visited him and he offered me some vodka. I was happy that somebody in this world still cared for me, that I was not alone. Slava suggested that I could stay at his place. I was glad to live with him.

Slava lived with his mother, younger sister, and grandparents. We had a separate room. Slava and I carried on our market business. Some time later I got a job as a real estate agent in the "Time Share" company. I used to hang around in the toy shop, searching for rich, well-dressed customers. As soon I spotted one, I encourage him to fill up the form. I handed the full forms back to the office.

Slava drank too much. He started beating me when he got wasted. I had to put up with it, I considered him to be a good man after all. He gave me a shelter.

One beautiful day Slava asked me if I would marry him. I said "Yes", even though he kept drinking and hitting me. The wedding was not flashy, we didn't even have rings. I was dressed in a white blouse and black pants. His mother arranged a party. We did not invite guests – we just had a simple family dinner.

Migrating To Israel

My grandfather – my mom's father, who passed away when I was thirteen – was a Jew. I found out that we could migrate to Israel. I shared this idea with Slava and went to Yaroslavl in order to persuade my mother to go to Israel. She was glad to hear it, so we took the documents confirming that my grandfather was a Jew, and went to the Embassy of Israel in Moscow so they could process our migration. Slava, my mother and myself were granted permission. When we applied for our international passports, I was told that I had to receive my father's consent for my departure to Israel.

My father lived in Kalinov. My mother and I boarded the train and went to see him there. After we had found his address at the inquiry office we took a taxi and went to his place. We found his house in the village and knocked on the door.

The person who opened the door was his new wife. She asked my mother, "Who are you?"

My mother replied, "We are looking for Pyotr. And who are you?"

"I am his wife", the woman said.

"I am his ex-wife", my mother replied. The woman let us in and hurried to inform my father that his ex-wife came over. My father was stunned when he saw us. He had not seen me since I was a little girl.

Mother said that we needed his consent so we can move to Israel. He did not want to sign anything, but his wife put pressure on him and he agreed. My father had a son from this woman. His name was Igor. I was happy to see my brother. He was couple of years younger than me. and he was surprised to see me too.

My parents and I went to the attorney and my father signed the consent form.

My father wanted to show us Kalinov so he took us to the seashore to collect some amber. There was a plant in Kalinov that produced amber jewelry. On our way back we were driving through the city. My father was so excited to see me, that he was nervous, and we ended up in the car accident. He hit a police car. My mother and I got out of the car and went away, leaving my father to sort it out alone.

We received the consent and went back to Saint Petersburg. The flight tickets to Israel have been booked six months in advance and we finally went to Israel.

In Israel

On 15th of March 1995 we landed at Ben Gurion Airport, and made our way to Netanya. Our aunt Mira lived there. We stayed at her place for two weeks before renting an apartment in Yoknaam. We studied Hebrew and I started searching for a job.

Our uncle directed me to a horse farm where I was hired as a groom. Since I was the only groom I had to look after twenty horses. I was walking from horse to horse without a break cleaning after them. Twenty horses! In Russia I had had to take care of five horses maximum, and I could ride all five of them. Here I was barely allowed to ride a horse. I was disappointed with the job. The stable keeper was a young woman. Slava told me it would be a difficult job for me, but it is good for the lady who keeps the stables. So I decided to quit the job.

I found another job at a printing office. My job was to fix the calendars after printing. One day the boss offered me some ice-cream. We had the dessert and he asked me to sit down on the couch. He wanted to have sex with me, but I turned him down. The next day he brought in another woman and told me I was fired. It was not easy to get a job in Israel. I started working as a hospital cleaner. I quit that job soon after.

Next I worked as a cleaner at the plant in Qrayot suburb. The workers there were Israeli, Arab and Russian. The boss was a lady, and she told me to clean the plant restrooms. When I started cleaning the workshop restrooms, Arabs started laughing at me. Our Russian men, who worked as office Autocad Designers, saw it and told me to stay away from the workshop restrooms, and to tell the boss that the Arabs wouldn't leave me alone. I complained to the boss and she appointed the previous worker to clean the restrooms. She made me clean the office. When I was cleaning the office, I had a talk with the Russians

I asked them "How did you manage do find a job as Autocad Designers?" They told me that they had graduated from the University and that I should study there too.

They told me that if you want a good job you need to finish university or an institute. Without a degree there's nothing to do in Israel. Even a simple secretary had a first university degree. I came home and told mother that I would apply and study at the University.

That night Slava came home drunk. He beat me. I locked myself in the bathroom. He crashed the door glass and started breaking up the door. I burst out screaming. The neighbors soon showed up wondering what was going on. I kept screaming and they called the police.

Slava broke the door, dragged me into the kitchen, took the ice out of the refrigerator and apply to my face. Soon the police appear knocking on our door. I opened the door and told them what happened. They took Slava and Me to the police station.

At the station we were interrogated and I was advised to go to the hospital and bring the documents testifying about the bruises on my face. I went to the hospital and brought the papers. They forbade him to go near my house, so he left.

Studying At the University

I took the documents testifying that I had attended secondary school in Russia and went to the University. The secretary looked through my documents and said that I'd only accomplished nine years of school education instead of ten (eight years in school and one year at a college). I needed to finish secondary school before entering the University, which required ten years of education in Russia.

The secretary said that I should go and attend a pre-learning course in University colledge. I went to the college and I was admitted to the one-year pre-learning course.

During the course I worked as a cleaner at the University faculty building. Slava called me, asked me to forgive him and come back. I agreed. Slava lived in a small room in the city center. I took my belongings and moved to his place. Slava's friend Andrei was married to my cleaning supervisor at the faculty building.

Slava told me how he had gotten drunk a few days prior. He got home and went to bed. He told me that suddenly there was a dead cat that jumped from the window to the bed. When he turned on the light there was nothing there.

"There he is, drinking to the blue devils!", I thought.

Meanwhile, I finished the training course, passed the exams and was admitted to the college, in the "Computer Programming" faculty. My boss at work decided to give me the cleaning supervisor position at the building of another faculty.

But Andrei's wife turned Slava against me for some reason. She told him that I slept with the boss and that's why he gave me the supervisory role. Slava attacked me again.

I said: "Let's talk to the boss". When we came to the faculty building Slava, Andrei's wife and I met the supervisor. I told him that Andrei's wife had said that I slept with him in order to get my promotion. Andrei's wife said that it was her, to whom he should have given this position. The boss denied this fact, saying that she can't be the supervisor at two faculties simultaneously.

At home Slava got drunk, grabbed the knife and assaulted me. I screamed: "Don't kill me! I will take my own life myself!"

I grabbed the razorblade and slashed my arm. Slava was shocked and put the knife away. I put a patch to the wound and left the house immediately. Then I went back to my mother's. I started the divorce process.

True Love

Back then I studied computer programming in the college. Essam, an Arab man who was twenty-six years old, was our lecturer on Window's applications. He was a bit plump, but well-built. He had long black hair that he tied in a knot. After seeing him several times I felt some spark in my heart. I realized I was in love with him. I tried talking to him on computers, coming up to him during the breaks and asking him to help me with my lab computer.

I felt that he was glad to help me; I could see that he got excited every time he saw me.

At the same time an Israeli girl called Segal began visiting him too. One day I walked into the computer room where Essam worked and I saw Segal waiting for him. I came up to

Essam and he was glad to help me. A flicker of jealousy ran across Segal's face.

Later, one girl who was Segal's friend asked me if I was married. I replied that I was, but in reality I was in the process of divorcing.

Segal quit the college. One of the tutors asked her friend "Where is Segal? Is she coming back?"

Her friend said: "Time will tell".

I didn't know how to tell Essam that I wanted to be his girlfriend. Normally a man is supposed to suggest serious relationships. I was afraid that he would turn me down. I wouldn't survive the shame and would have to leave the college as Segal had. I kept my love secret. I told no one about it, nor even my college friends, not my mother - no one.

Two years later I had finalized my divorce and started working on my college project. Realizing that my time in college was nearly up, I became very nervous that I wouldn't see Essam again.

I told my mother about my love. I shared my feelings with her. I felt awful, nervous and I cried a lot. Mother said I needed a doctor. I agreed. I went to the doctor and told her about my affection. I got hysterical when I was telling about it. She said Essam should know about it.

I plucked up my courage and went to the college. I came into Essam's lab and told him I wanted to speak to him. He walked into the corridor and I asked him if I could be his girlfriend. He smiled and replied politely that he already had a girlfriend. If I had told him a year ago, then he would have agreed.

Burning with resentment I walked away. What could I do back then, two years ago!? If he had turned me down, I couldn't have finished my study! Why hadn't he told me himself?

Meeting Yigal

I was searching for a job some time before graduation. However, I still had to defend my thesis and introduce my project. Even after graduation it was still difficult to find a job. All employers wanted to hire first degree engineers from the University, not practical engineers like me.

My mother's friend Dov decided to introduce me to his acquaintance Yigal who helped him with computers. He said Yigal was the one who could help me find a job. I said that I wanted to show him my project. We set-up an appointment at Dov's office.

After installing my project program on the office computer I waited for Yigal. The door opened and the man of twenty-five, skinny, with a bald patch on his head and a briefcase in his hand entered the room. We sat down at the table. I showed him my project. He said that the program was very good, but the display resolution support had to be added.

Afterwards we had a conversation in Dov's office. I told him I was searching for a job and that it was difficult to find one. If he had connections in the companies where he had worked before and inquired about a job for me I would be grateful. I asked him where he worked at that moment. He said he was finishing his aeronautics doctor degree at the University. After our conversation he gave me a ride home. That's how my friendship with Yigal started.

I was in a bad mood after Essam's rejection. I decided to share it with Yigal. I came to him and told him about my unrequited love for Essam. But still I did not lose my hope. I called our tutor Eti who knew Essam. She used to work sometimes in his lab. She said that Essam really wanted me to be his girlfriend before; I should have told him earlier. She added that now I had no chance to get him back.

I needed to make up three copies of my project for the examination committee. I asked Yigal for a printer and he brought it to my place.

Since I had no friends I decided that Yigal could become a good one. But just a friend, not a lover. We started going out. One evening we went to the seashore. We were sitting at the pub drinking piña coladas, my favorite alcoholic drink. Afterwards we went for a walk on the beach. There was a district of hi-tech "greenhouses" by the seaside. We saw a 'Microsoft' logo and Yigal said that one day I would be working for this company.

We met a second time at the Haifa's Bahai temple. I wore a black dress and black high-heeled shoes. We went down the Louis Promenade and everybody turned their heads when they saw me. I am a gorgeous girl, I felt. Yigal was proud to walk with a girl like me. We came up to the fountain; Yigal put his arms around me and asked me to be his girlfriend. I didn't need it, since I was crazy over Essam. I told him we would stay friends, but nothing more.

I still could not stop thinking about Essam, so I decided to talk to him one more time. I went to the college and found him in the computer lab. I came up to him and said that I wanted to talk. We went outside. I lit a cigarette and told him hysterically that I wanted to be his girlfriend. He said that if I had talked to him a year ago he would have accepted my offering. He mentioned my boyfriend but I was divorced. Even if I had had someone I would have dumped him.

I cried. I begged him to leave his girlfriend. I told him that she didn't love him as much as I do. I said she wouldn't beg him the way I do. He asked me how I knew that she wouldn't. Puffing cigarette smoke at him I cried that I love him and hate him. He said that I shouldn't drive a car in this state. I said I would catch a bus.

I went away, with tears showering from my eyes. I went, no matter where, couldn't see the road, stumbling over stones and walking through sand. When I got home I decided to commit a suicide. I walked from one drugstore to another, buying sleeping pills. I bought enough medicine so I could take all of them at once and fall asleep forever. I lacked the courage, so instead I lay wrapped in a blanket for days on end.

Yigal called me and told me his mother had found a job for me as an office secretary. I wasn't ready to work as a secretary. I was qualified as a programmer. I said that I didn't want to be a secretary. Yigal raised his voice and started yelling at me through the phone receiver.

"Madam, it is not the right way! You've got to go for the job interview!"

I was shocked - Yigal was yelling at me. I hung up the receiver. I told my mother that Yigal yelled at me, mother said: "Yell back at him".

I saw yelling at people as inappropriate, so I called him back and told him to come here and take his printer back. I said that I didn't want to have any business with him. Yigal came over and took his printer back.

One day later I was heading back home. There was a rose hanging on the door handle. I thought that this one was from Essam, but mother told me that it was Yigal who had left this rose here. I got really mad and threw the rose away. I didn't want to have any more to do with Yigal at this point.

One day Dov told me that Essam was getting married. While walking downtown I saw an advertisement of a fortuneteller who could see the future using cards. I decided to go to the fortuneteller and to find out about Essam.

I came to her; the lady placed the cards on the table and said that Essam had a baby, so I should quit pursuing him. I decided not to search for him anymore.

Working as A Programmer

Eventually I found a job as a programmer in a company producing industrial scales. I asked for just the minimum wage because I really wanted to get the job. The company was located far from Qrayot district. They arranged transportation from another company for me.

Meanwhile I defended my thesis publicly at college and got one hundred points for the defense.

After half a year of working there I was given a huge project for a poultry slaughterhouse. The work was very intense. We even worked on Saturdays, during weekends.

I got the job of designing a terminal for the cash registers. This work should have been given to a team of programmers. My boss did not know exactly what I was doing but tried to explain to the manager that she was in control.

One day the manager told me that my transportation expenses went beyond all limits. I decided to rent an apartment in the district of the Qrayot, which was closer to my work. Our financial worker picked me up in the morning. He turned up the music as loud as possible. We went to pick up other mans from Acre on the way. Those men were noisy and they were shouting and yelling in the car. I couldn't stand such noise. Later I understood that loud noises play a pivotal role in my illness.

As days passed I sat in my room crying and thinking about Essam. One day our selling agent came to me and offered some arak. We drank arak, talked for a while and I went home.

On my way to work I heard a song on the radio. There was a phrase: "It's hard to be without you and I'm not meant to be with you, when I say that I don't love you, you know I'm just lying". It seemed to me that Essam must have asked to put this tune on the air especially for me.

At that time, we moved to the poultry slaughterhouse building and my work became even more intense. I worked so hard on Saturday - at the end of the week that I got the icons in the menu of my program all messed up. I found it strange, how could the icons get all messed up!?

I decided to call Nir, my teacher. I wanted him to come to my workplace and give me feedback on the program I was making. I called the college but he was unavailable. He was having the classes at that moment.

At the same time, I was involved with Jehovah's Witnesses in those days. After work my mother came to me and waited for Dov to give us a lift to Haifa, so that she could go home and I could go to the meeting with Jehovah's Witnesses.

I had a strange feeling. It seemed to me as though everything happening to me had been scripted long before. Dov came. I took the Bible, and then we went to Haifa. There was a small fan that looked like a helicopter in Dov's car. He pointed a finger at the fan and I realized that we were being watched from above. Dov dropped my mother and me at her house and left.

I came to my mother's place, stayed there for a while and started getting ready to go out. Mother kissed me goodbye, like she would never see me again. I went outside and headed to the meeting with Jehovah's Witnesses. Walking down the street I was afraid I would get shot from above. I saw a girl walking down the opposite side of the street, hair long and white just like mine, I decided that she was copying me on purpose, so that those watching confused us.

When I came into Jehovah's Witnesses' room I saw Tamara, a girl of my age. We had met before. She told me with understanding; "Thank you for coming", as though she knew what bothered me. She was giving a lecture on the stage.

After the lecture a man came up to me and said: "Come over again, if you can".

Tamara, her friend and myself went to the bus stop. It was Friday and the street my mother lived in had been blocked for religious purposes so we had to take a detour.

"It is strange that it happened in the street where my mom lived not somewhere else!", I thought. We came to the bus stop and Tamara asked me if I had the money to pay the fare. I took out fifty shekels, tore them and threw away. I said that money meant nothing. Tamara picked up the money and gave it back to me. She said that I would need it to pay the fare.

The next day I came to our department and asked the poultry slaughterhouse-programming manager to give me the job here because I didn't want to work in Qyaiot anymore. He said that there was nothing he could do about it. He already had enough workers.

The next morning, I decided not to go to work. The financial worker who had been picking me up in the morning called me, and I said that I would stay home. I looked out my window. There were two cars parked outside with American flags on them. "OK", I thought, "I'm invited to America".

I was hungry so I went outside and decided to go to the nearest store to buy something to eat. A man on a bike started following me; there were wooden boards in his sack. He scared me and I popped into the nearest store. The cake looked nice and I decided to buy it. I realized that money has no value and I was about to leave without paying, but at the last moment I left twenty shekels for the store clerk. The store clerk took the money and gave me no change. I took a walk in the park. There was a pregnant woman walking in the park. I started following, as if I was protecting her. When I noticed that she didn't need my protection I started walking through the park.

Then I saw a man carrying a document case. "That is the job for me!" I thought. The man got into a car shaking the case and drove away.

"It is strange", I thought, "Why didn't he give me the case? Maybe I should have asked him for it?" I sat down on a bench back. I felt exhausted and broken.

A man with his girlfriend stopped next to me, the man said, "Water?" I shook my head meaning "No".

I came home broken and exhausted, took a glass and broke it in my room. Then I took the mop, mounted it and started hopping on it trying to take off and fly. But the mop wouldn't take off so I threw it in the closet.

Suddenly the telephone rang, I picked up the receiver. It was my mother. She said "You broke something and hid something in the closet, just like a little kid, just like a little kid". I got scared and hung up the receiver. How could my mother see what was going on in my room?

There must have been hidden cameras somewhere! It means that my mother belongs to some secret organization! I felt panic attack. I found Essam's number in the telephone book and called him. A girl picked up the receiver. I asked for Essam. The girl said he was at the studies and she asked who I was. I said that he knew me.

Then I called Tamara and told her that I was going to come to the Jehovah's Witnesses meeting with my leopard dress on. I suggested meeting and she said: "Come to the meeting, and then I will come".

I called Yigal. I thought that his previous job was somehow connected with the place I work now. I wanted him to help me, since he was studying at the University at the aeronautics faculty; I wanted him to make me a spaceship so I could fly away.

When Yigal answered I asked him where he had worked before. He said that he had worked in the district of Qrayot. But I was too exhausted to ask him about the spaceship. Yigal did not know why I was calling him and he was quite aloof towards me because of our bad relationship.

I decided that Microsoft would soon take over the world of programming and threw the "Microsoft Access" book into the rubbish bin.

I decided to go to Haifa, I did not know why. I went outside, came to the bus stop and saw bus in the parking spot. Even though it was a bus I got in without paying the fare. There were soldiers sitting inside. The woman behind me said: "The girl is brave". The bus went in the direction of Haifa. As it was reaching Haifa I didn't know where it would go next. I decided to go where the bus goes. The bus arrived at the central station of Haifa.

I got out of the bus along with the soldiers. I went down to the first floor of the central station and started walking around with no idea where I should go next.

Suddenly I saw Dov with my mother standing in line for a bus. I came up to them. They were surprised to see me there.

I asked my mother "Where are you going?"

She said that she was going to Riga to her mother. They left the line and walked aside to talk to me.

Dov asked me "What do you do at your work?" I said that my job was to fix system bugs and that there is not a single system bug that I could not fix! My mother asked me why I wasn't at work. I told her I didn't want to go to work. Mother insisted – I should have gone to work. I just laughed in response, but mother didn't. She said "Go to work!"

Meeting the Devil

I came back from Haifa in the evening. I went outside to buy cigarettes. Suddenly an SUV stopped in front of me. The door opened, but nobody came out, as though I was expected to get in. I looked inside. There was a girl and somebody else sitting in the car. I could not see the girl's face, just her shoe. The shoe was gilt. I wanted to get into the SUV, but then I thought that it would be stupid to get into a strange car. I stepped aside. Soon I realized that I was being followed. I raised my hand, as though I was trying to relieve those following me. The SUV, as well as two other cars, drove away. I went home. I did not expect a call from my mother. She said she wanted to pay me a visit. She asked me if I wanted her to bring me something. I asked her to bring some tomatoes. Soon

I forgot that mother was to come over, I was thinking about Essam. I waited for him to come.

I was lying in my bed when somebody rang the doorbell. I thought that it was Essam and rushed to the door. But it was just my mother. She came inside. She didn't laugh. She put the tomatoes in the fridge and asked me why I didn't want to go to work. There was something strange about her behavior. Her eyes! Her eyes were dead, it seemed as there were no soul in her body. She started dialing some numbers on the phone. Somebody answered. She said that her daughter didn't want to go to work. Somebody told her something in reply and she hung up the receiver. I laughed.

"What are you laughing at?" she asked and hit me on the head, looking at me with those dead man's eyes. Now it was not funny at all! She threatened me! She sat down at the table, took out the cheese and the sausage and put the knife in the middle (The Jewish traditions forbid eating meat together with dairy).

"Oh, she's got a knife!" I thought. I panicked and asked for Dov's number.

I called Dov and told him in Russian, "The pig came here to eat". I asked him for help and said that I wanted to live. But Dov understood nothing and hung up the receiver.

"What do you want from me?" I asked. "When were you born?" she asked me in response. I was born on December 31st 1974 on New Year's Eve, which comes after Christmas. At that moment it was 1999. If you turn the nines upside down, it will make 666; Satan's mark!

As soon as she finished her meal she told me "Take your clothes off and go to bed!" I stripped to the skin for it was really hot and lay down in bed. She also took everything off but her underwear and lay down in bed with me. Horror was filling me. I tried to run; I stood up and tried to open the door. I found out that the door was locked and she took the keys out and hid them. I had a feeling that she wanted to kill me.

"Go to bed!", she ordered. Trembling with fear I lay down in bed.

As I tried to fall asleep I heard a gurgle in her stomach. As I opened my eyes I saw a mass of filth flowing out of her stomach and a snake crawling out of it. "This is the end!" I thought. I jumped out of the bed and I tried to jump through the window to get out of here, at least go somewhere else.

Mother followed me, she gripped my hand. I punched her in the face and jumped through the window. I fell on my back. I landed on the first floor roof from the second floor. I saw my mother shouting through the window "Geula, Geula..." Leaping back on my feet I rushed to the drainpipe. I climbed down the drainpipe from the roof down to the ground, leaped over the gates and ran down the street screaming "Satan! Satan!"

The people from the neighboring house saw me standing outside naked and brought a blanket and a chair so I could cover myself and sit down. They called an ambulance. I was afraid that my mother would get out of the house and keep pursuing me.

They asked me "What happened?" Pointing at the window I jumped on my feet and screamed: "Satan! Satan! My mother is Satan! I escaped from Satan!"

The paramedics took me into the ambulance. Then my mother came with my clothes. She wanted to accompany me but I wailed in horror, "Don't let her in. She is Satan!" The paramedic didn't let her in the car, however they took my clothes. The car started out leaving my mother behind. I felt glad that I was finally free and not in the locked room. I put my clothes on in the car, still I had no shoes. The car stopped and I was told to get into the other ambulance car. I got into the other car and lay down on the couch. The car was driving somewhere.

Suddenly I saw several men standing above and looking at me. I thought they were doctors. A bearded man of fifty leaned over me. I told him that I had escaped from Satan. He said "I know; we were there too". I asked "Who are you". He answered "We are Angels".

I lost consciousness for a while. When I opened my eyes again, there was nobody in the car but the paramedic and the driver. "Where are they?" I asked.

"Who are you talking about?" the paramedic asked me.

"The people that were there" I answered. "There was nobody here but me and the driver" he replied. Then I realized that those were the angels. They saw everything and they helped me to escape from Satan.

The car stopped. We arrived at the Bloom hospital in Yoknaam. The medic gave me a hand and helped me get out of the car. I walked down the corridor barefooted and saw my mother staring at me with her dead eyes. Quickly I ran past her.

The nurses showed me the room where the doctor was sitting. I was screaming "Don't let her in here!" I told the doctor about what had happened that Satan got into my mother's body and I jumped out of the window. I wanted him to believe me and told him just to take a look into her eyes! The doctor understood everything, nodded his head and asked me "Maybe you want to go to Tower?" ("Tower" is mental hospital in Yoknaam). I asked them to take me anywhere just to avoid meeting my mother again! The doctor asked me to wait in the corridor.

As I was sitting in the corridor it seemed to me that the end of the world came and I was going to go to heaven. I was called outside where the car was waiting for me. When I got into the ambulance car the driver asked me "Do you know where we are headed?"

"To Essam!" I said. "Essam is my friend!" I said thinking that the end of the world already came.

"To Essam!?" said the driver "It's Tower where we are going to". On our way to Tower the driver told me "You will stay there for just one night and they will let you out tomorrow, there's nothing to be afraid of".

When we got to Tower, I had to wait for the doctor. There was a board on the wall that said "Pay Attention to Suspicious Objects". Then they led me to the "Emergency" department. They gave me pajamas and took blood samples from my veins, then led me up and down the corridor.

As I was walking down the corridor I looked through the window of the door leading outside and saw my mother sitting in the corridor beneath the "Pay Attention to Suspicious Objects" board. "She is the suspicious object!" I thought. "Don't let her in here!" I screamed. "She is Satan!", I shouted.

"Don't worry, we won't let her in here", the doctor said, trying to pacify me.

I was sitting on the floor for there were no chairs around. After sitting there for a while I went to bed feeling relieved that my mother wouldn't be let inside and that I'm under the protection of this facility.

I woke up and went to the canteen for breakfast. I ate an egg, drank kefir, then I came up to the window and tried to close it, but I could not. "The windows are opened and can't be closed! Windows!" (meaning "Microsoft Windows") said I.

Suddenly I saw a cemetery across the road through the window. "Surely it is the end of the world!" I thought. "Now all the dead must rise!" I saw an old lady sitting in an armchair, took her hands and tried to help her stand up, but for some reasons she wouldn't stand up. A nurse came up to me and told me to leave the old lady alone.

The doctor called me into his office and asked me if I knew where I was. I wanted to say "Heaven", but I collected what was left of my mind and said "In Tower".

The doctor asked me what I did for a living, where I worked, which city in Russia I had come from, and if I had health insurance. I told him that I had come from Saint Petersburg and that I had been selling clothes there. After telling my story of Satan once again I sat silent. The doctor told me he was transferring me to the eighth hospital department. I didn't care where I went, as long as it was just away from my mother.

Hospitalization at Tower Mental Hospital

The male nurse took me to the eighth department and left me waiting at the department threshold. The door shut behind me. I was scared to meet my mother, as soon as I entered the department I fell down on the floor at the door screaming "Satan! My mother is Satan! Don't let her in!" The nurse, whose name was Dima, helped me to get up and soothed me, he said I would be safe there. I was brought to the ward and Dima gave me an injection. My mind grew dim and I was panting for breath. I staggered down the corridor trying to hold on to the nurse station window.

Time was passing by and I can't remember exactly what was happening to me back then. I remember one morning when I woke up and saw my ward mate's husband came to visit her.

Her condition was not so well, she started pulling her underpants on her head.

I got acquainted with my department neighbors. I met a girl who had set herself on fire. She scorched her forehead and hair after she saw that her husband had hung himself. I became acquainted with a man whose name was Ramsey. He said that he had a brain tumor.

I was given pills. I didn't know their names. In the morning they took a blood sample. My mind grew even dimmer.

In the nurse station I decided that Doomsday had already come and that all people must walk around naked like Adam and Eve. I tore my pajama dress off me and stood naked in the station. The station was glazed and Ramsey saw me through the station glass. "OK, mans, tie her up" the nurse said. They grabbed me and led me to the ward. They dressed me in pajamas, a diaper and strapped me to the bed. Everything was like in a fairy-tale. A female nurse came into the ward. I said that she was Alyonushka, and I called the male nurse Dima Ivanushka (the names from Russian fairy-tales). Then another nurse with a blue nose looking like an alcoholic entered the ward. I asked him if he drank vodka. He told me that he didn't. Then a fat nurse came into the room and I told her she had a pig snout.

The next morning my condition got much better and I didn't want to tear off my clothes anymore. As I woke up I saw Dima wearing black and looking at me. I told him that I was hungry, he unstrapped me and I went for breakfast.

One day I saw Dima standing at the nurse station. He was applying medicine to the wound of the girl who had set herself on fire. The doctors came in. Dima said that the doctors arrived, but I grabbed him by the hand and went out screaming "It's my doctor! It's my doctor!"

"I'm not a doctor" said Dima "I'm a nurse". Dima told me "Don't jump from the window again you can break your neck".

One beautiful day I saw my mother walking down the passage. Her eyes didn't look like the eyes of Satan anymore. She was an ordinary woman. The nurse came up to me and said that my mother had come to see me. We sat down at the table. I tried to distance myself from her as far as possible so I could spring up and run away if something went wrong. I asked her how she knew I had broken the glass and hidden the mop in the closet when she called me and said "You broke something and hid something in the closet, just like a little kid".

She told me she hadn't called me and hadn't told me that. She told me that when she had come to my place she had called the hospital and told that her daughter did not want to go to work. She was told to wait until next morning and see what happens. "If she still doesn't want to go to work, then take her to the doctor".

"If I knew that you're unhealthy, I would have taken you to the hospital at once" she said. I relaxed a little bit now. My mother didn't have any eyes of Satan anymore. She brought me the slippers; I was still walking barefooted. When she left, I threw the slippers away into the rubbish bin and said that I didn't need anything from her, but the nurse took the slippers back from the bin. She said I was going to need them soon.

The pills made me drowsy. The doctors asked me to talk about what had happened. I walked into the room where all the doctors were sitting and told them my whole story in a worried manner.

Meanwhile Ramsey started courting me. We were talking and walking together. He was at the open department and I was at the closed one. Every evening at 8 pm after taking the pills, we could walk to the opened department, as they did not lock the doors.

But one evening Ramsey didn't come up to meet me as usual. I found him sitting in front of the TV. I asked why he didn't come up to me. He said that the doctors had forbidden getting close to me.

I was still making attempts to contact Essam. I found his number in the phone book and called him. A man picked up the receiver. I asked "Are you Essam?"

"Yes, I am Essam" answered the voice.

"Have you given lectures at the University?" I asked. "No, I have never given lectures at the University" answered the man. I didn't know what to say so I hung up the receiver.

In my department I met a girl, Valya. We knew each other from college. She joined us the last semester. "Valya, is it you?" I asked her, "We met in college, do you remember?"

"Yes, I do" she said. "What happened to you?" I asked her.

"I felt sick at the college and I voluntarily went to the hospital".

One day after the hospital knitting lesson all the patients had a one-hour break. I stayed alone with the teacher as I was infatuated with my work. Suddenly she took out the lighter and lit it. She was a non-smoker. I thought she was trying to set me on fire, so I fled from the room in horror.

"Are you Scared?" asked Valya sitting behind the door.

I was thinking about Essam and I realized that I had to talk to him first. Trying to find some help wherever I could think of, I called our former college teacher. I said "Hello, Nir, it's me, Geula from college, remember? The long-haired blonde. I'm in Tower right now. Could you come over and see me?"

"Yeah, I remember you, you were looking for me recently, but I was at a lesson. I will come over" he replied. "I am at the closed department number eight" I said.

One morning the nurse came up to me and said that there was a guest who wanted to see me. I walked out of the ward and saw Nir. We sat down at the table. I told him the story about the snake coming out of my mother's stomach. He was shocked and scared.

I told him I loved him and wanted to be his girlfriend. "I've got a girlfriend" he said "but you were in love with Essam" he said.

"Essam is a maniac and I've got no friends" I replied bitterly. "You will have many as soon as you get out of here" he said. He seemed to be scared and left in haste.

Valya came up to me and said with respect: "Nir himself came to see you!"

Afterwards I remember that in the past, when I got to work by taxi, I asked for tax receipt so I could get my money back. The Hebrew word for "ticket" was "kabala". Somehow the expression "Give me the kabala" engraved in my memory. "Why on earth do I always ask the cab driver to give me the kabala?" I thought.

One day I wanted to see my doctor. We sat down in the armchairs and I told him "Satan stole God's kabala". The doctor understood and nodded his head.

One day a social worker came up to me and asked me if I wanted to get a social insurance. I didn't understand him so I said, "I did not want to retire; I wanted to get back to work". This is because most of the retired people get social security insurance.

Next day a girl named Alisa came up to me. She investigated the patients' condition, and she asked me to take a computer test. I agreed. They tested my ability to think and answer the questions within a limited amount of time. There were different cards and shapes on the computer screen. They changed fast. I had to click on the identical cards. When I finished the test, Alisa said that my results were the highest she had ever seen.

My mother called me and asked me if I wanted her to bring me anything. I said "Heavenly water". "Heavenly water" was the name of natural water brand. When mother came she gave me a bottle of "Naviot" (another brand), I got angry that it wasn't "Heavenly Water", I shouted at my mother and told her "That's what I'm going to do with your water!", and poured the water into the rubbish bin.

Time was passing by and doctors make the decision to transfer me to the open department. As a test they let me into the open department in the daytime.

Walking around the open department I saw men shaving with sharp blades. I thought they wanted to cut me to death, so I pulled a towel on my head so they could not recognize me. The nurse saw it and offered me a pill, but I screamed that it was a poison! The nurse said that the doctors should give me the pills and brought me to the closed department.

Some time later I was eventually transferred to the open department. There I met a girl called Miri. We were in the same ward. One day when we were lying in bed Miri shouted at me. She said she was Satan herself! I got scared and rushed out of the ward. One woman advised me to complain to the doctor and the doctors came for a round. I told them that Miri scared me and that she had shouted that she had been Satan! The doctor said that Miri would be transferred to the closed department.

The doctors allowed me to leave the hospital for one day to see my mother. She brought my clothes. I tried to put them on. The jeans got too tight. I put on a few pounds during my staying at the hospital because of the medications. I pulled the jeans on with great effort and was ready to leave the hospital.

We went to Dov's office. Mother worked there as a cleaner. I asked for a glass of water and mother gave me one. But as she was giving me the glass, she disappeared somewhere. The glass magically flew into my hands. "Wow! The glass goes into my hands without any assistance!" I was scared. I went to the kitchen where I found mother cleaning up. I told her I didn't feel well and that I wanted to go back to the hospital. We packed my things and I got back to the hospital.

I told the doctor about this accident and added that working on Saturdays is forbidden (according to the Jewish religion). "Why? We work on Saturdays " the doctor told me.

Mother came to see me from time to time. She brought yoghurt.

It is important for the normal people to understand the human experience in the hospital. Most of the patients, nurses and doctors are heavy smokers. This is the way that most of the patients pass the time. This is the only thing that gives a lifting experience after being dozed off from the medications. The patients are treated as second class: most of the times their complaints are ignored by the nurses and doctors because of the possibility that the patient's requests could be hallucinations or psychosomatic.

Walking in the ward you could see patients whose hygiene is fair. The patients are doing odd things like urinate on the surroundings, rather than go to the restroom. When the time for meal comes they rush to the dining hall and eat two portions of food getting fat due to the medication's starving side-effects. The patients in the ward are kept because no suitable drug is found. This means that most of time they are not feeling balanced and coherent to function and perform basic tasks. This abnormal atmosphere usually comes as a shock to visitors.

Time was passing by and I spent four months at the hospital. There was no hope for recovery. The doctors didn't want me to go for ECT (Electroconvulsive therapy). They were afraid I would forget everything I had studied in college. They tried to balance me out with pills.

One day the doctor asked me to come to his office. We started talking. I asked how he could explain the fact that I had seen Satan. He said it was hallucinations (dreaming wide awake). I asked how he could explain that my mother had called me and said that I had broken something and hid something in the closet. He said he had no idea. The doctor told me that there was a testing of a new medicine called "Iloperidone". It should help me. He offered an agreement for me to sign and so I did.

All the fears were gone; I can not say I was 100% healthy but I was at least well-balanced. I didn't want to go home. I was afraid to see my mother so I asked the social worker to find a hostel room for me. The social worker said that it would take much time to wait for the hostel room and would be better to go back to my mother's house. The doctors told the same thing adding that I should not be afraid of my mother.

The doctors advised me to get a social insurance so I could receive 1800 shekels (about $500) a month. Once I found out about it I went to the social worker. He told I was offered this before but I refused. Now I wanted to get this insurance. The social worker said all the necessary papers would be prepared and sent to the Social Security Agency.

Life After the Hospital

I was discharged from the hospital and came back to normal life with my mother as soon as the doctors agreed that I wouldn't be able to live alone. Mother said that she had taken all my belongings from the house in Qrayot where I used to live and canceled the rental agreement.

I got the social security insurance and began working as a cleaner at a clothes store. It was hard to find a job as a programmer. Dov tried to contact the company in Qrayot where I worked but they didn't want to talk to him.

Meanwhile, I got fat. One day somebody knocked on the door in my house. I opened the door, it was Yigal. He came in; he wanted to get my computer to back up the data. He took it and went away. A few days later he gave the computer back and I found out that he had deleted my project. I wanted him to explain himself. Dov had said that I didn't need that disk.

I quit the cleaning job and began working at the jewelry store opposite my home.

I was searching for the programmer job and finally I got a call from one company. They invited me in for an interview. When I came to the interview I showed my project to the employer. He asked me where the database was. I told him that there was no database in my project. He said he would discuss it and if I was the right person for the position he would ask me to take an exam; he also told me that I would have to work with the "Visual Basic" program. I had no "Visual Basic" so I decided to ask Yigal for it.

I called Yigal and asked him if he could give me the "Visual Basic" program. He told me to come over to his place to take the program. I came to him and we had a talk. I didn't mention the fact that I had been in Tower. He gave me the program and asked me if I wanted to be his girlfriend. I agreed.

At home I installed the program and realized that I know nothing about the database, so I decided not to go to the exam. When I got the call I cancelled the appointment.

Yigal suggested that I write a program for "Windows CE" for portable computers. Yigal brought a palmtop and I started writing the program.

My bank sent me the PIN code for my credit card. I put the papers on the shelf without any suspicions. Meanwhile my mother invited me to the restaurant. We went to Mount Carmel and had a dinner. A few days later when I looked at my bank statement printout I found out that all the money had disappeared! I remembered that I had left the PIN code on the shelf. My mother had stolen my money from me! I came up to my mother and accused her of stealing all of my money! She didn't deny it. She said that we had had dinner at the restaurant and she needed money anyway. I couldn't inform the police about it, for I was depending on her.

I worked and could save some more money. My mother decided to buy an apartment in the district of Hadar in Haifa. She got the loan from the bank and once everything was sorted she asked if I wanted to move with her to the new apartment. I gave her 7000 shekels for refurbishing otherwise I would have to stay in the old apartment. I didn't want to be alone.

We moved to the new place and every month I paid my mother 500 shekels for residing at her place.

One day Dov asked me if I wanted to move to a kibbutz up north and gather fruits for living. I refused. Yigal said that he heard Dov talking to my mother about that. My mother said there was a "goat" in her house that took too much space. She wanted to get rid of me. Yigal said they wanted to send me to kibbutz in the north of Israel. There I will definitely be killed by Hezbollah's Katyusha rockets. I got extremely mad at my mother and Dov.

By that time, I had finished "Free Hand" and "Photoshop" college courses and started searching for a job. I found an advertisement in local newspaper that some hotel required a reception secretary, so I called this hotel. Manager told me to come for an interview. There he told me I would undertake a short training course and start working part-time. Since the social security insurance didn't allow me to earn more than $500 this job suited me perfectly, so I started working at the hotel.

One day Yigal came to pick me and my mother up. He saw my mother beating and pushing me while getting into the car. He said he wanted me to leave my mother and move to a place of my own in Neve Sha'anan district. He would help me with the rent. I felt happy that I would finally get rid of my mother and in turn she would be happy to get rid of me.

She helped me to pack my stuff with great pleasure and I moved to Neve Sha'anan. She called me on the cell phone

Yigal had given to me. She wanted to come and collect the keys from her apartment. At that moment I was at the hotel, she could come anytime and get them. Shortly after she came and took her keys.

Yigal invited me to go to Eilat, a resort town in Israel. We packed our things and went to Eilat by plane. At the evening as we were walking down the pedestrian path I confessed to him that I had been at Tower. Yigal knew, Dov had told him. Yigal said he'd been finding out what I'd been up to all this time.

I had been working at the hotel for two years already and it had been four years since I left Tower. During this time, I came to Tower from time to time for the pills. Once they decided to cancel the drug Iloperedone since it negatively affected the heart and the medicine hadn't received approval from the Health Ministry.

From that moment on my health got worse and I started hallucinating. I was given another medicine. Later on I had panic attack. I called Yigal and asked him to take me to the hospital. I had stayed in the hospital open department for a few days before they prescribe me Resperidal 2 mg. pills. Then they let me go home. Meanwhile I went on a diet and lost 85 lbs.

During the time I worked, Yigal was giving me a ride to the hotel and picking me up after.

One day my boss told me he was going to go on vacation. He wanted to appoint me as the supervisor for this period. My task was to collect the money and store it in the safe. I felt a great pressure then.

One day Yigal's mother came to pick me up from work. I felt my mind darken and I couldn't control myself.

My landlord raised the rent; I didn't want to pay more so I started looking for a new apartment. I read a newspaper advertisement that one old man with a dog was letting a room. I thought it suited me so I contacted the old man. His name was

Aaron. When I came to him he said that he was looking for a woman who would live with him and take care of him, apart from that he required $250 a month for residing. I decided to rent the room.

I was totally confused and I couldn't get a clue what I was doing. I lived at Aaron's and spent time at Yigal's. He lived in the district of Denia. I started to hear a voice in the apartment. I didn't exactly take care of Aaron. I myself needed somebody to take care of me. Aaron got angry with me and said that he wouldn't sign the renting contract. He told me to get out of his apartment. He did not wait for me to leave before he invited other women to see the apartment.

Soon I found another apartment in Nave-Sha'anan I packed my belongings and moved there. It was too far away from the hotel. I couldn't afford getting there on my own so I quit the job.

I decided to adopt a dog. I wanted an Afghan hound, but thoroughbreds of this kind were very rare in Israel, and it was impossible to get a puppy. Then I went to the dog pound. I saw a dog at the entrance. It resembled an Afghan hound but with a thin coat. I asked the pound workers if this one was Afghan. It was Afghan mixed with Labrador. I took this one. I called her Daphne. I signed the dog adoption documents and took her home. The vet doctor told me I should give Daphne a rabies vaccine. I came to the clinic, there was a man named Mark. He suggested placing a chip in her. After all, chipping and vaccination has been done I paid $150. Mark gave me his business card. I did not exactly know what I was doing. I started visiting Mark at the clinic for no reason. Daphne began snappy; she sat down on the bed and refused to climb off. I called Mark and said that Daphne bit me. I asked him to come and see what was happening. Mark came over and chased

Daphne off the bed. Then he recommended giving her back to the dog pound. I felt pity.

As I was walking Daphne down the street a mad dog ran past, trying to bully us. I unleashed Daphne. Daphne ran after the mad dog. I lost sight of her and went home, then I called Mark and said that Daphne ran away chasing the mad dog. Mark told me to go outside and look for her in the vicinity. I went outside and found Daphne near the house.

Afterwards, Yigal said that I should find my father and invite him to Israel so I won't be alone after my mother didn't want to take me. I called the inquiry office of Russia and found my father's telephone. I called the number and a man answered. It wasn't my father, but a person with the same surname. I told that I was looking for Pyotr Salamonov living in Village.

The man said that he would find my father and hand him my telephone number. After a while I got a call from my father. I just wanted to be sure that it was my true father I asked him what he had brought me when I was a little girl. He said it was a doll.

"Correct" I answered. I asked him why he had not paid alimony when I was a child. He told me I had been hidden from him. I asked him to come to Israel. He wanted to come, but he needed an official invitation from Israel.

I went to Tel Aviv to the Russian embassy. I explain that I wanted to invite my father. They sent me to the Ministry of Internal Affairs of Israel.

On my way back to Haifa I heard two women talking. "He helped you, give him a gift" one lady said. I thought that it was addressed to me. I decided to buy Mark a goldfish as a present. When I got out of the train I went to a pet shop and bought a goldfish. I gave Mark the gift. He checked if the fish was healthy and then put it in the fishbowl.

I returned home from Hadar. That day there was a litter disposal worker strike. Litter laid everywhere on the station.

Taxi cab stopped next to me and the driver invited me in. I hesitated. I looked at him and at the litter, back at him again and then at the litter. He shut the door and drove away. The bus had arrived in Nave-Sha'Anan. I had a walk not far from Mark's vet clinic. Suddenly that taxi stopped by my side and the driver said: "Hey, litter! Litter!" He scared me so I rushed into the clinic and told Mark the taxi was haunting me. Mark went outside but the taxi has already gone.

At that time there were terrorist acts in Israel. Suicide bombers blew themselves up in buses.

Yigal's mother took me to the shopping center. I decided to dress like a policeman. I bought grey pants and a blue shirt.

The next day I went to the Ministry of Internal Affairs in Haifa dressed like policeman. There was a long line there, so I crossed my arms standing in line and began protecting those standing in line with me. When my turn came up the door shut in front of my face. The security man who let the customers in said "Those who work in security, come in". He let me inside. When my turn in line for the secretary came up I told her "Abba to Israel" (Aba is the Hebrew word for 'father'). I wanted to say "Abba" for reason. There was a connection between the name of the "ABBA" band and my father. The secretary told me that my father could come to me as a tourist.

I decided that black is Satan's color. I collected all the black clothes I had and threw away in the bin outside.

I had a regular check in hospital. That day the doctor decided that I am psychotic and insisted on hospitalization but I didn't want to. I had a dog and I couldn't leave her. They changed my prescription.

One day I and Yigal went to Home Depot and I noticed that all the prices are ending in 99.9 I got scared and told Yigal and said that this is the sign of the Satan.

I was afraid someone would break into my apartment and steal my pills so I bought a small safe and hid my pills in there.

I considered digits 3,6,9,13 were Satan's digits and 1,2,4,6,8,10,11 belonged to God. I made up a password not containing those digits.

Back then I suffered from backaches. I went to the doctor and he gave me the pills for osteoporosis. I was taking the pills and locking them in the safe.

I felt bad and Yigal took me and Daphne to his place in Denia. I was sleeping in the morning when suddenly a voice told me "Go to Tower". I dressed up and went to Tower with no questions.

The Second Time in Tower Mental Hospital

I arrived to Tower, bought a pack of cigarettes and waited in the Emergency department. They finally let me in and I changed out of my clothes to pajamas. The nurse asked whether I wanted to commit suicide. I said I did and showed her the scars on my hand I had since the incident with Slava.

I was transferred to eighth department. I met a girl, Marina. She was sitting on the floor smoking. She asked if I am a lesbian. I said no and sat down opposite to her.

Sometime later, I went to the nurse station and saw the nurse Jakov. His parents were from India. He reminded me of a doctor I knew.

I asked him "Are you Doctor Gov?" He denied. But the resemblance was terrific. Then I offered him to go to the hotel with me that I use to work for. He refused. I saw the gilded silver ring on his finger. I wondered if he wanted to be my boyfriend. He said he was married and showed me the ring. I thought that engagement ring could not be made of silver. I started running after Jakov.

Yigal decided that he is going to take me as a "project" and try to do the best he can to "heal" me or at least take care of me. From that moment on my life changed for the good.

I called Yigal. I asked him to look after Daphna while I am in Tower. He arrived to the hospital straight away. I told him I need medicine for the osteoporosis. He asked doctors for the pills, but they said I could not take any medications, but psychiatric. Yigal was not happy with the answer because he knew that the nurses and doctors would deny any request.

Yigal asked where I kept my pills. I said "In the safe". He wanted the security number. "Oh, you want a number! I will give you then 11, 2, 4, 2, 11". I named the combination of

God's figures that I created. He returned back shortly and said it was incorrect code.

"Now you want a number! All right, I will tell you" So I told the actual code and he brought me the medicine. There was only one pill. I thought there was no point in one dose so I threw it away.

Once in the nurse station where I was taking the pills I asked Dima, "What disease I am suffering from?" He replied "Paranoid Schizophrenia". I became close to Marina. When she was sitting on the canteen floor having a meal I sit next to her having mine. She had liver hepatitis and recently the doctor said she had got AIDS. That was not an issue. We remained friends. I said I was sent by Mossad, she said she was sent by Shabak (Israel Security Agency).

The pills had very bad effects. I was torn apart. Doctors insisted on Electro Convulsive Therapy but I rejected it because I was afraid. I needed to do electroencephalography to know what is happening to me. I was afraid of that too. When a nurse took me to the room, I saw the girl sitting on the chair. She had suction pads with wires attached to her head. I was scared to death; it might be very painful so I started screaming. Doctor said, "It is not painful look at the girl, she is sitting still"

After the EEG has been done, I returned back to the ward. I told everyone I had ECT (Electroconvulsive Therapy) but the doctor corrected me. "That was just EEG, not ECT". After that I felt energy streaming out of my hands. I took other people's hands and they could feel the electric waves. I proclaimed myself a Bio-Energetic.

Yigal visited me from time to time, he brought me cigarettes and "outside food" like pizza so I'd feel better and not just have food associated with the hospital.

I went on chasing Jakov. Marina and I were sitting on the floor next to the nurse station. I crossed my legs and was turning my head in Indian manner looking at him. I asked Yigal not to visit me. He never came back. But I needed smokes so I called my mother and let her know that I am in Tower. She brought me cigarettes. We just had a short talk in the corridor – I was still a bit scared after our first meeting in this hospital. I asked her to go away. I wanted Yigal to come. He was glad to see me again.

One day I passed by the nurse station. I noticed the reflection of a man in the window. He was about 35 years old with long curly hair, big eyes and Roman style outfit. I approached to the window but nobody was there. I thought: "Satan himself. He put me here and came to visit".

I had spent 4 months in the clinic with no progress. Yigal did not want me to stay there any longer. He contacted my doctors asking permission to transfer me to the private clinic. They rejected it. The reason was I was not ready to live the closed department and require ECT.

One day I was standing by the open department door. I was waiting for the moment when the nurse opens the door so I could rush through. I managed to break through but I fell down. I was taken back to the closed department. Next day the nurse took me for a walk in the hospital. Afterwards I returned back to my department. Yigal also had the permission to take me outside. We had a short 15 minutes walk and he confessed he took Daphne back to the pound. I was upset. I complained to Dima with tears in my eyes, bud he just suggested I take another puppy later on.

At that time, Marina was subjected to ECT. She needed 12 procedures. I told her I needed it too but I was so afraid. She assured me it would help.

The nursing personnel treated the patients like animals. I could not breathe, I clutched at the windows and walls, I shouted, "Help! Please help me". Nurses advised me ECT. I thought that Red Bull would give me wings and I would fly away from here. I asked Yigal to bring me Red Bull but nurses took it at the entrance because it was the alcoholic version.

At the station, I saw Dima, Jakov and other nurse. I said Dima and Jakov that they are angels. Then I advised the third one to drink Red Bull as it will be helpful. He poured a drink that Yigal brought in the glass and handed to me. I was about to make a sip but the nurse took it from my hands saying "Look at her, she would have drunk it!"

We had a new patient – a tall man with beard. I told Yigal about him. He looked like Jesus Christ. Yigal agreed. The man really reminded Jesus.

Dima took our department for a walk in the garden. I planted a peach pit, hoping to see the tree someday. Dima was sitting on the bench. I felt a sudden rush of energy. I did a somersault and sat under the tree singing the songs by the band "Mirage" to Dima.

I climbed the tree looking for an exit but I could not find it. The other man helped me to climb down.

We had lunch in the canteen. Everybody was eating slowly; I did not want to wait. I noticed the hole in the door lock so I tried to pick it with my spoon. The door opened. Nurses were surprised. They called doctors who wanted me to explain myself. I did not want to return back to the canteen so I showed them how I picked the lock later on. They left me alone but made a note to everyone to lock the door properly.

I felt very bad. When I passed through the nurse station my mind darkened. I grasped the wall and crawled on the floor. Nurses suggested having some rest. I thought I was dying. ECT was my last chance to survive. I asked for it.

In the same time Yigal was trying to do the best he could to help me. He thought that because Iloperidone has stopped to be administered to me my health deteriorated. Yigal was trying to find a medicine for me. Since the doctors stopped giving me Iloperidone and other medicine had no effect, he was trying to study the molecules of the medicine using the "Hypechem" computer program. He read different articles in pharmaceutical scientific journals. When he did not succeed in finding such drug he contacted the "Novartis" pharmaceutical company that developed Iloperidone but they could not help him because it was harmful to be used anymore.

Yigal at that time decided I should be treated by Dr. Tal, a private psychiatrist, rather than the doctors at the hospital. He thought that the closed department was very depressing for me, even though I was not well yet. The interaction with the other patients and the closed department would be depressing by themselves.

He prepared a document for me to sign saying that I wouldn't like to be hospitalized here and treated by the doctors at the hospital, but with a private psychiatrist. I signed the document. The doctors at the hospital that were probably offended by this move asked Yigal for a talk. All the doctors were sitting in the room and try to convince him not to release me from the hospital. Yigal said that he preferred that other doctors would treat me because my requests are reasonable and are not answered. That there had been no success in the treatment I was getting and I was just confined in the closed department. Yigal persisted and said that Geula do not want ECT to be performed on her.

The doctors told Yigal that I would be released as soon as he asked. Yigal left. The nurse called the doctor immediately and soon I signed all the necessary papers for ECT. I was not myself.

Next morning the nurse gave me the injection. "I should not be afraid of the ECT", the nurse said. But the medicine had no effect. When they came for me, I hid behind the curtain screaming "You are going to kill me!"

The morning after Dima called me "Geula. ECT." I trusted him and I agreed to go. The doctor checked my teeth - they could crash during the procedure. I lay on the couch; they put a rubber band on my head and administered the anesthesia. I could feel the faint electric current rushed into my head. I lost consciousness. When I woke up I heard noises in my head. On my way to the ward I could not recall what was happening. I had ECT 3 times and it made me feel better. Perfect I would say.

Yigal came to see me. He was not pleased that I had the ECT in contrary to the agreement with the doctors. I asked him what had happened, why and how long I am here. He told me that I came here myself and had spent four months there so far. Doctors promised that my memory would be restored.

One morning Dima walked the patients from our department to the canteen. On the way back I confessed I would marry him. He said he would agree if I did not have a boyfriend.

I recovered. They transferred me to the open department. Dima said goodbye to me and Yigal adding, "See you in another century. Do not get here anymore!"

The social worker offered me to sign up for the "rehabilitation package" in Social Security Agency. They would help me to find a job and give the accommodation. The apartment is much better than a hostel but social workers will come to see me regularly. Once I was told, I am to clean the apartment myself and it did not worth the trouble.

They also asked me to tell my story to another social worker. The lady came to Tower and I tried to tell her about how I met Satan. It was difficult. There were long pauses in my speech.

Once I heard the voices of my mother and Dov. The nurse asked me whether I wanted to see them. I did not want to. I ran outside just to stay away from them. During my time in the hospital, Yigal was visiting me regularly, but mother came only once.

Yigal arranged a private doctor for me. I would be doctor Tal's patient when I left Tower.

As I was being discharged from the hospital doctors said to Yigal: "Look at her now and remember how she was before getting here."

I was prescribed Risperdal 2mg. After discharge I was living in Yigal's place in Denia, waiting for the apartment near Neve Sha'anan. I felt great.

I had a call from a social worker. There was a lady in Nave Sha'anan who was looking for a flat mate. I went there to have a look. This room was smaller than the other one but the price was the same. However, I moved there. The social Service found me the job as a programmer in "JTE Software".

At that time, Yigal was finishing the thesis for his Doctor's degree in the faculty of aeronautics in the University. He wanted to move to the USA when he got the degree. I needed the tourist visa and Yigal said that I would need a driver's license.

Schizophrenia patients usually do not have a driver license mainly because of that fact that they cannot afford a car on their social security annuity. They also mistakably think that by taking the psychiatric medications they are not allowed to drive. I filled in the form at the DMV office and was asked to be interviewed by a special committee. I came to the interview and was asked which medication I am taking. I told them and they approved to allow me to learn to drive. I started learning to drive and soon enough I graduated the course and got my driving license.

The landlord made us clean the apartment. My flat mate had a bi-polar disorder. Every night she turned the stove on and went to the bed. We had huge electricity bills to be paid. Then I kept switching it off after her. Once I turned the boiler on to take a shower. She turned it out. It was annoying.

"The idea that two mental patients live together was not a good one", thought Yigal. One's odd behavior triggered the others and added conditions of tension and pressure. I left the apartment and moved to Yigal. Afterwards we moved to his mother's place.

Yigal tried to find cure for my illness in non-conventional treatments. Yigal got acquainted with doctor Weisman. He was doing the Native American Studies as well as acupuncture and Whole Hearted Healing. I was attending his therapy sessions because it was to heal my schizophrenia. I had to go through the emotional traumas in my life and fight them mentally. As for me it was delirious and I called him a shammer. He laughed at me.

I went to their office of the social worker and explained myself that I didn't want their help any more. I remained silent when they asked me the questions. I said I am self-reliant enough and feel much better with Yigal help. I wanted to leave the apartment they gave me. They agreed to leave me by myself without interference.

The therapy sessions with Weisman were over. He said I had recovered and I could stop taking pills if the doctor allowed. I did not trust him. Schizophrenia cannot be treated.

I rented another apartment in Neve Sha'anan, and got an American visa. Yigal finished his doctorate and decided to search for a job in the USA. I moved to Yigal's parent's apartment and quit my job. Because the job at "JTE" software company was introduced by the social worker it paid only $500. I spent $120 on transport and was left with only with $350 after taxes. I got more in the hotel, working less. I got the temporary accommodation in Yigal parents neighbor's place. We were to move to the US soon.

Living alone in that place I was crying. I said to Yigal that I will never have an Afghan hound dog. Yigal promised me to find the puppy on the Internet and assured me I will have an Afghan dog. I stopped crying and happiness engulfed me. Soon we found one in Netherlands. It was red haired black masked. We contacted the kennel and they said it was the last Afghan in the litter. We transferred $1000 immediately and waited for the puppy to arrive. Finally, I saw black eyes looking at me from the box at the airport. We took him home. I was glad I had a true Afghan. I called him Chavi.

Once I found Chavi whining. He hurt his paw somewhere.

At that time Yigal found a job in Albany, New York. He said he would go two weeks earlier than me. He wanted to settle down there, find the accommodation, and buy a car so I would go after him when everything was done.

Yigal and his father had gone. I stayed with Chavi packing the bags. Yigal called me after two weeks as he promised. Everything was sorted out so I took Chavi and left Israel.

Living in The USA

Yigal met me at the airport and we went to Albany. He was doing his postdoctoral in RPI. I felt very well. I created an account on My Space and had doves on my main page. Doctor Tal reduced my dose of Risperdal by half a milligram.

After six months' time Yigal resigned his job. He had disagreements with the management. He soon found a new one and we moved to St. Louis, Missouri. I had the tourist visa so we had to reapply for a new one every six months.

American food made me fat so I decided to keep to a diet. I wanted to be in touch with Dima from Tower. We called Yigal's mother and asked her to get Dima's contacts. She found him. He did not work in eighth department anymore, he moved to the children's department. Yigal's mother gave Dima my contact information and he sent me an email. He never wrote me though. All I got from him were pictures. He sent me animals and nature images.

I lost 110 lbs and decided I was looking good. All I needed was the treatment from acne. I got some pills and vitamins making sure that on the label it did not have side effects and would not affect my schizophrenia. It was entirely natural product. Despite my carefulness, this was soon to be the wrong pills to take.

Trip to Las Vegas

One day Yigal offered me to go to Las Vegas; we got tickets and booked a Time Share Hotel. We were walking down the casinos, taking photos and then decided to see the Grand Canyon. We arrived to the Grand Canyon by bus. I wanted to have the horse tour round the Canyon and we went to the Ranch. I saw a real Indian in the ranch where we got the tickets. We had a tour round the Canyon and went to the restaurant afterwards. The Indian drew a face of an Indian on a stone. I heard the voice behind me "She is good for the "strip"". The Indian sent a reproachful look to the person who said that.

We returned back to Vegas and were walking on the main streets when I had a sudden fear attack. I heard someone said, "She will escape! She is from Israel" After a little while the lady who passed us by hissed "Dump this mad woman and bring us real Geula!"

I was waiting for Yigal at MacDonalds. I heard one girl said to another "You won't have children. You will live forever!" I walked downstairs to find Yigal. The woman with kids said, "Bring children!" I said to Yigal that I was unwell and wanted to return to the hotel. I spent the rest of the day in the hotel room while Yigal was playing in the casino.

We were driving Yigal's car and stopped for a while. I noticed a girl in a short black skirt walking down the pavement. The man from passing car whistled and another said "Look, she is a woman-snake!"

Woman-Snake

On my way to the airport, I was scared. I heard someone said, "Essam made a big mistake!" How did they know about Essam?

Yigal left me sitting on the bench. Suddenly one man said "Snakes are everywhere!" One woman with two children who was staying next to me pointed a finger somewhere behind me saying, "Woman-snake is there!"

She left her children and went away. We boarded the plane. The woman behind me said, "You are a bitch and we have a sting!" Another man added, "Do not look in her eyes! She will scare you!" I heard the voices everywhere "Keep the windows open!", "Do not sleep naked!"

Now, it was clear to me. I understood that Satan created the women-snakes promising them immortality. I also thought that they were not able to give birth. They had a sting in the underbelly. They attacked the other women infecting them. It takes time when the snake gets the brain through the spine. The woman can be saved during this time. Otherwise there is only surgery operation that can take the snake out of the brain. The woman-snake hypnotizes the normal woman, making her undress so she could not flee. Then the woman-snake attacks the normal woman. That is how they multiply! "My mother was a woman-snake!", I thought. All these thoughts hurtled in my mind.

We were waiting for our luggage in St Louis airport. I heard a man voice saying "She will own her clothes, her credit card and her house". I knew he was talking about the woman-snake. We got the luggage and went outside. I heard someone said, "Get married! They'll get your body!" How do they know me?

The Third Stroke of Schizophrenia

Yigal was not home. I heard the voice from upstairs; "Do not drink milk!" I took the milk and drank it purposely.

"She hears us!", whispered the voice.

Later on I scanned my pictures and sent them to Dima. He said I looked awesome. I made a phone call to Tower.

"Hello" said a male voice.

"Can I please speak to Dima?"

"It is me" he replied.

"Its Geula here". I told him about Las Vegas but did not mention the woman-snake.

"How do you feel?", he asked. I said I was not good. "What is the time there?" he asked. I said it was nine o'clock. I felt sudden fear again and told him that I would call back.

I told Yigal that I wanted Dima to come to visit us. I sent him greeting cards and also an invitation. I threw away the photos that we made in Las Vegas. After that there was a voice from outside "Maruska screwed up!" I realized I made a mistake. I went outside and took the photos out of the rubbish bin.

I was lying on the sofa. I felt horrible. I heard Marina said: "We are coming to you!".

"Marina! Is it you?", I said aloud. I heard the noise in the stairway that scared me. Yigal found out that I was unwell and called Doctor Tal. She ordered to increase the dose of my medicine. My mind darkened. I took Chavi and went outside. I was walking straight aimlessly and I noticed a helicopter above. I thought it was chasing me. But the helicopter did not land so I continued to walk. I saw a bank building and entered it with the dog. I was offered a chair there. "Call the ambulance please! I do not feel good" I said. They got me a taxi instead.

I told the cab driver to get me to the nearest hospital. I got to the Board Hospital. The front desk person said that dogs were not allowed here. Then I lied that I was blind and the dog was my guide. They asked what I was complaining at and where I was from. I said that I did not remember. They put me on the sofa and attached the suction pads to my breast. I had to release Chavi's leash. He laid still for a while and the suddenly rushed outside. I ran after him. When I found him and returned back. The doctors said I needed MRI. They thought I had lost my memory. They will look after the dog at the meantime.

I was angry. "What MRI are you talking about? I need to go to a mental hospital!" The doctors were surprised "a mental hospital?" They asked me about a contact person. I named Yigal.

I heard the noise of propellers. I thought that Dima and Marina are coming here by the helicopter. Then a lady in military uniform entered the room. I wanted to be taken by her.

"Take me to the asylum!" I screamed.

"Dogs are not allowed in the asylum!", the nurse replied. I threw away the glasses in the bin. Yigal came over shortly and took me home. They had found his name in the telephone book.

I thought I needed to go to a mental hospital; if I was in Israel they would have taken me there immediately! Yigal took me back home. I did not know what to do and how to get to the hospital. I was walking around the house when I heard a noise in the stairway.

I went to the door to have a look when the voice ordered "Jump!". Without questions I jumped out the window. I jumped from a height of two stories. It was lucky that we were living in the second floor and not higher.

I was lying on the grass with my leg broken. I heard Marina's voice "Dima is coming; Dima is coming". But Dima did not come.

I saw Yigal approaching me. "I will get the blanket", he said. I hopped on one leg to the car. The door was open so I got inside and signaled. I called Yigal but he did not turn up. I signaled more and more before he came. He took me back to the Board Hospital. They made an X-ray, put the bandage and took me in the ambulance to the main department of Board Hospital. I thought they should have done this earlier. Yigal followed the ambulance car. They took me to the emergency department and made an encephalography. Yigal said they have doubts where do I need to go: Psychiatry or Orthopedic department. Then I rushed outside hoping along leaning on the chair. I screamed: "Take me to Israel! Take me to Israel!" So they sent me to the Psychiatry.

I lost my consciousness. I found myself in the closed department. The only thing I could remember was that there were orthopedists that came and attached the plasters to my leg. They took a CT scan to find out what was wrong with it. I had no clue what was happening. They asked me how much Risperdal I took.

Yigal visited me. Soon I was transferred to the open department. Orthopedists said I needed an operation, but changed their mind later. I had a talk to a nurse called Tom. He said the acne pills caused the stroke. I said "But there were only natural ingredients!" Tom explained that these pills were to speed up the metabolism so in turn it caused the schizophrenia stroke. My normal dose of Risperidal was increased and I was discharged. Mental hospitals in the US do not keep the patients for the long time. It is expensive.

Another Meeting with The Devil

I was lying on the sofa at home. I could hear the voices of two men upstairs. They talked nonstop. I asked who they were. They said they were wolves. I could not recollect what exactly they were discussing; some nonsense. I could hear the noise of the hammer crashing wood. It was a neighbor doing his weight exercises.

One man said to another: "Will talk on the telephone". Another replied: "Yes. Bye!" Chavi barked and I heard the man walking down the stairs.

"Satan will live here!" he said as he approached my door.

"Satan! Satan again! How many times must I escape from Satan!", I thought. "If I keep running away from the devil, it will be a real Hell!" There was the noise of some car outside with the sound of heart beats. I could not get up and have a look. I thought it was Satan's vehicle.

Then I heard a lady's voice from above. "Why is Satan chasing you? He must love you!" I told: "Come here, Satan! Let's talk!"

I addressed to the devil in the mind's eye "What do you need?"

"Your heart!" he replied.

I closed my eyes and saw a hand giving me a rose made of plastic. "Take it if you want" said Satan ", but sorry, it is made of plastic".

In the evening I heard that Chavi was barking. Two ladies talked again. "Hit the skull and skull will crash!" She was speaking Russian and everybody there were speaking Russian. Then she asked me: "Do you want to ride Satan's car? You won't keep up with your crutches! Do you know what car does he have? It rides fast so cops cannot get him!"

At night, I saw the car light. I thought the car came after me and I began untying the bandage. I could not get outside though. My leg got twisted and I could not move it properly.

I thought there was a gang hiding by my house. I looked at the window and saw cars parked nearby. There was nobody in the cars but I thought the gangsters were hiding. "Wait for me in another life!" I said.

The voices said that I have a radio transmitter implanted in my leg. I asked how it is possible. They replied that it is in the plaster the orthopedists put on my leg.

I was lying in my bed and casting the stars to the space. Suddenly a female voice told me to stop it. That was a bad sign. There were important people talking in space.

I felt like I was dying. The voice of the nurse from Tower. said: "Are you going to die? Go to the hospital immediately!"

I asked Yigal to take me to the Board Hospital. There were many people in the emergency department. I was told to wait. I did not have patience and I went outside and got into the ambulance car that was parked nearby. The guard told me to leave the ambulance. I went back to the second floor.

I saw a couple from India. I told them I did not have a home and asked if they want to take me with them. They said something and went down the corridor. I followed them limping. There was an office behind the glass door. I was sure it was Satan's office, and he will come soon. The Indians sat there for a while and then left.

"They left me alone" I thought. I went down to the first floor where guards met me and took me to the emergency department.

They wanted me to sit on the wheelchair as if I could not walk. "I can walk!" I screamed and hit the nurse with the crutch. They laid me on the sofa and put a harder bandage on my leg. I spent an hour there. When I saw Yigal he told me that he lost me and thought I went home. He did not find me there and returned back to the hospital. I was sent to the open psychiatric department.

Meeting Malcolm

I noticed a man about 50 years old with good body, long black hair and grey temples. I thought there was Satan himself. Finally, we met. I felt I was in love.

Doctors tried to figure out what was happening to me. I refused to talk. They said I was not in a hotel and I had to tell them everything.

It was boring. Yigal bought me an iPod and I asked him to upload songs by the Russian band "Mirage", Dana International and some paintings by the artist Boris.

I showed the paintings to nurse Tom. There were: the girl with dragon, the girl kissing snake and many others. I confessed I have been haunted by Satan for nine years since my first schizophrenia stroke.

I showed the pictures to Mal and ask him to save me from Satan. He just said it was an artwork and the pills will save me.

Then I showed the paintings to the doctors. I said there were gangsters in my house and they can read my mind. Doctors offered me an ECT bur warned it may cause epilepsy. I refused.

I was lying in my bed and listening to the voices above. They were talking nonsense. But suddenly a new female voice addressed me. "Never jump out of the window! Keep the door open instead". I knew it was the guarding Angel. Indeed, why should I jump out of the window? It is handier to use the door.

Mal was a head nurse in the department. He had a privilege to prescribe medications. He gave me Atevan and I felt better.

I was in love with Mal. I told him he was looking like Israeli singer Zvika Pick. I asked him if he is Jewish. He was. His mother was from Latin America.

I saw the nurse shuffling cards. She always had clubs. "All right. Clubs are doctors, Spades - Satan's people, Hearts – the ones who fight Satan, Diamonds – the rest of people." I decided to pick only hearts if I wanted to fight the Satan. The other patients invited me to play with them. I collected only hearts and won the game.

I wanted Mal to know that I love him. I gave him my business card with phone number but he did not take it.

One night I felt remarkably awful. Everybody knew about me. "You will get it!" said the voice from the television. The voice spoke Russian. One patient said "Russians are already on air!" I was ashamed. I asked the nurse for a pill but I could not remember which. The nurse went through my papers bud did not get it for me. I was suffering the whole night and in the morning when Mal came I said: "Jesus Christ, Crucify me also!" I complained to yesterday's nurse and he gave me the Atevan.

One night I came to Mal and he gave me his hand. There was a golden ring with engraved imps. "Here is Satan!", I thought.

I was taking the shower and threw away the golden chain that Yigal gave me.

There was a new patient in my room, her name was Mary. She believed in God and always had a Bible. She said she also heard the voiced and she was subject to ECT. I persuaded her not to do it – it will cause epilepsy. I told her about the gang that chased me. She said they were demons.

I had a talk with Mary. I said, "If the demons exist, God exists too!"

Mary picked up the earphones from my shelf. I thought the voices could come from it.

I felt much better and doctors decided to discharge me. I wanted to give Mal my business card and I wanted the craft teacher to pass it to him.

On the day I was to be discharged, I had breakfast in the canteen. Mal came over and said: "I will be your nurse today" He stroked my hair and I was so glad. I said: "Go to Hell!" He gave me injection of Respirdal. I offered a hand but he said the needle were too big.

Yigal came to pick me up. I got dressed and we left the hospital.

Crazy Days

I stopped taking my pills as I thought they were poison. I was lying in my bed and heard Satan's car coming. It was approaching with a sound of heartbeats. I heard someone upstairs played the songs by "Queen". Some minutes later I heard the voice of a little boy: "Queen?". I was proclaimed a queen! Satan had many queens everywhere.

The female voice said "He visits his lovers while their husbands are at work! The neighbors will gossip that you have a lover!"

I asked the voice: "Who are you?". It replied: "We are your doves." I had doves on my website. I was terrified and called the police.

When policemen came, I asked them to take me to the Board Hospital because I was scared. They said we were not going to Board Hospital, but they would take me to the "Saint

Mary" which was nearby. The police called the ambulance and I was taken to Saint Mary hospital. The doctor asked what pills I took. I said I was taking nothing, as it was a poison. The doctor gave me the pills and took me on the wheelchair to the corridor. The taxi was waiting for me but I did not want to go home. I was afraid of demons. I wanted someone to give me a shelter. I laid on the floor. The nurse took me to the couch in the corridor.

I watched the girls passing by and I begged someone to take me. "We need your money and then you can get out!", I could read their mind. Nobody wanted to take me so I got the taxi and went home.

Yigal was working daytime. Dima did not email me anymore and I told him he was mean. He dumped me in time of need. I bought earrings on ebay. I put them on as soon as I got them. The voice from above said: "The AIDS transmits through the earrings!"

Chavi barked and the man walked down the stairway and said:" Get used to your husband!" In the evening, Yigal was watching the TV. There was a church chorus singing something. I heard Satan was singing, "I have AIDS, you have AIDS". I was scared to death. I thought I was sick and asked Yigal to take me to Saint Mary to check me for AIDS. It was the night time. Yigal made a wrong turn and soon the police car appeared. They forced us to pull over. The policeman said we had not stopped when he signaled. Yigal explained he was in rush to take me to the hospital. The police car accompanied us to the Saint Mary' door. At the front desk, I told the nurse that I had got the earrings on ebay. I might have got infected. "A little chance", she replied.

I waited for the AIDS check but nobody came so I decided to return back home. I told Yigal I wanted to date Mal. I called him using the department code that doctors gave to Yigal. I asked for Mal and the voice replied "Mal is speaking."

"It is me, Geula, did you received my card?" "Yes I did". Then I asked him out. He rejected. He said he was married. I was upset.

"He is not allowed to date his patients" – I told Yigal – "But if he knew that I am not in the Board but in Saint Mary it would change everything!" Yigal knew I was psychotic.

"He is married; you cannot do anything". He told me to take a medicine but I did not want to.

I bought the golden ring and engraved, "Geula and Yigal are friends". I put the ring on and said, "We will stay friends forever".

I heard the voice of my college friend Anya. She said, "I am talking from IBM. We sent you to kill Satan but you fell in love with him!" The man was walking down the stairs saying: "We will be back as soon as Satan turns up". I thought: "Chavi heard them as well, he would not bark if he did not hear them!"

There was a woman who said, "What you will do with him? Nothing!"

Later on, I heard the woman screaming. One man said: "Lets help her!" Another one replied: "It's too late, she has already pricked her". I realized that woman-snake bit her.

I was scared to stay home alone. The woman-snake one could come after me. Therefore, I took a knife and began walking with a knife in the apartment.

I was in my bed at night. The women went down the stairs. They said "Geula, we apologize for being noisy. When Geula leaves the apartment here will be light of candles ". How did they know my name? There were probably hidden cameras in my apartment.

I told Yigal I was the Heaven Ambassador, because I was born on New Year's Eve night after Christmas. He said he was the same. He was born on 9th of Av month. In the Jewish calendar it is supposed to be the date when the Jewish Messiah should be born. Yigal always took my words seriously and respected me, not like the rest of the world.

I heard the voice of my youth friend Valeria, we went to the stables together. She said she was chased by demons. "Go to the clinic" I told her.

I decided it was the time to get rid of the bandage on my leg. I called the ambulance and headed to the Saint Mary. The X-ray showed that my leg was not good enough. So the doctors cut the cast and applied the soft bandage and released me home.

I felt bad that night. I called the police and said I needed the doctor. They called the ambulance and I went to Saint Mary. I asked the paramedic if he knew Mal. He did not. I was taken to the psychiatric department. I was also asked about my contact person. I named Dima from Israel. I screamed I had AIDS, I was asking for a check. The doctor came to see me. I saw him in Board Hospital. He said I needed an extra Risperdal. I laughed saying I did not want it.

Next day I saw Valeria or the girl who was looking alike. I asked her out to have a horse ride to the Grand Canyon. She smiled but did not reply. I joined her over the breakfast and asked her name. Her name was Sarah and she came from Latin America.

I got rid of the bandage but I was afraid to step. I leaned on the chair and slowly walked the corridors.

I tried to call Mal but he was not in the hospital.

I had a roommate in the hospital. She said she heard the voices and put cotton pads in her ears. She asked me if I heard them and what were they telling me. I said they were talking nonsense. I recommended her stop putting cotton pads in her ears, otherwise she would go for the ECT.

The doctor said I am going to be discharged. They needed my address but I did not want to go home. I did not have Yigal's contact. I said I was homeless. They sent me to the homeless asylum.

I did not have crutches. When I got to the homeless asylum, I was given two crutches but one crutch was broken so they gave me a wheelchair. To find a bed I needed to get up the second floor. I said I could make it. They took me upstairs. The building was probably 200 years old. There was an altar in the middle of the room. I asked the nurse to call the Board Hospital and inform Mal that I was a homeless.

This was a women's asylum. We had a dinner, prayed and went to beds. Demonic voiced got to me even here. The hammer banged somewhere above. I was wondering, why I was here, Yigal was looking for me! I went downstairs and demanded to be sent home or I would call the police. She called a taxi. When I came home I was glad to see Yigal, he said he lost me.

Next day I decided to go to Kalinov to see my father. I could not find my passport. I took my Russian one that was expired and went to the airport. It was early morning there were no passengers around. I came to the security and asked if I can go to Russia with my expired passport. He took me to the security station. During the investigation, I said I had schizophrenia. They demanded papers from police and the hospital. I asked for the ambulance to get to Saint Mary. The ambulance car took me to the hospital. The doctor gave me the paper with the diagnosis "Depression". I went to the police. I asked the driver to wait for me. I could not find the address of the police department. I was so tired. I went home.

I asked Yigal where my passport was. He said the police took it. I asked Yigal to take me to Mal. I took the lighter that I bought on ebay for him and we went to Board Hospital. We call Mal at the front desk and he came down. "Geula!" He smiled. I said I loved him and gave him the gift.

"Drop it", I thought he would throw away the lighter but he did not.

"Who is it?" – He said pointing at Yigal. "He is for security" I answered. Mal asked did I go to the Board Hospital. I replied something like "Oh, Board! I am in the Saint Mary Now!" Mal left and we went home.

Later on, I began to hear the voices from everywhere: from watches, from dog figurines, cat figurines, and from my golden Griffin. I put all that in the rubbish bin. The noise ceased. When Yigal came home he took the dog out of the bin and placed it on my table. He spent the night by my side.

When I woke up, I saw Yigal holding the figurine in his hands. "He wants to kill me with it" I thought, and called the police. When the police arrived, I explained that he wanted to kill me.

"What did he do to you?" the Policemen asked. I replied: "He took the figurine and tried to kill me".

"Did you take the knife?" the policemen remarked.

"What knife? I took a cigarette!", I took a long cigarette out of the box.

"Look how he parks our car!" I said to the policemen and pointed to our car in the parking spot.

His car was not parked properly. "Nice try!", he replied.

I heard the voice of the girl-snake that was in love with Satan. She was somewhere opposite the house. "Satan is mine!", she shouted. "Go to Israel. We have enough of Queens, go away or you will kick the bucket".

We began to converse telepathically. There was another voice of a neighbor woman. "I cannot bear it. I will kill her". But she never did.

Satan came to the house above ours, where they got together: Satan, Girl-snake and their friends. I decided to go see what was going on there. I walked around and went into the house. I saw it was a funeral home. I thought they were having a meeting in the hall. I heard a voice of the nurse from Tower close to the house. "Is it you, redhead?" I asked. She was somewhere nearby talking nonsense.

"Boil the potato" I heard a woman's voice from the top. It was late at night, Chavi was barking and I heard a man say: "Chavi".

How did he know the name of my dog? In the morning, I heard the voice of another woman from the top. She said: "Do not be afraid when they come after you. Get your things ready".

I packed up a bag and went up to the top floor. I knocked on the door. A Chinese man opened the door. I entered the apartment and said I needed a shelter. He did not understand anything and closed the door.

I went to Edward's apartment; he was my dog-lover friend. He opened the door. I said, "I need a place to hide". He said that he was sick and shut the door. Suddenly, the police came and ordered me to get back down to my apartment.

I saw a man coming out of the house carrying a large suitcase. I thought, "There must be a camera". It was the daytime; I was sitting on the balcony. I smelt kerosene coming from the top. I saw a girl coming out of the house. I called the fire brigade. A huge fire truck came over soon and firefighters entered the apartment.

"Where did you feel the smell?" I pointed up. They climbed to the second floor but found nothing. I told them about the lady but they did not understand and left.

In the evening, I was lying on the bed and listening to the conversation between two men. They said "She thought we were two robbers but we are two imps! We will get the money from her but what to do with the engineer?" I got up and walked out the door, but still I could hear them. I went to Yigal and asked him to listen to the conversation. But Yigal did not hear anything.

Next day Yigal and I went to Burger King. I had a burger but suddenly I was scared that "Snake could be transmitted through food". When I got home, I felt something in my stomach. I thought I was bit by a woman-snake.

I called 911 and said: "There is strange body in my stomach". Soon a fire truck came and the man asked me to get into it. I went through some check and was told to call the ambulance. An ambulance came over and took me to the hospital. At the hospital I was checked again, they gave me Maalox (stomach medicine) and sent home.

The next day I was taking the bath with flavored powder. Strangers were passing by my door. I heard "We spiked the sperm". I jumped out of the bathroom and threw the powder away.

Lying in bed, I could hear the voice of the boy: "The Bitch conceived!"

"What does this mean?" I asked mentally. "Something good" the voice of a woman replied. After a while, I heard the voice of a child in my stomach. He talked all sorts of nonsense.

"This is a child of Satan" I thought. "He is in the stomach and chatting already! It is odd enough".

"Salt! Give him salt" said the voice of God. I bought a pregnancy tester but the tester showed a negative result. The voice of the child in my stomach continued chatting.

The voice of Israeli nurse told me "Do the hair, make up, get dressed and go to your Mal". I got ready and went to Mal. I arrived at the department and called Mal. "Yesterday I was bitten by a woman-snake and now I'm pregnant" I said.

"Who's the father?" he asked.

I wanted to say "you" but I said "I do not know. I was spiked with the sperm".

"Go to the Emergency" said Mal. When he left, I lit a cigarette. The nurse came and asked to retain from smoking.

The security came later. They checked if I had brought weapon. Then they said: "Get out of here and do not come here anymore or you will go to jail".

I went home by taxi. When I got home, I said to Yigal that I left the car by the hospital and we need to get it back. We got a taxi and brought the car.

Next day I decided to go to Board Hospital because I felt bad. There was a huge line and I screamed "I am crazy! I am crazy!"

The guard took me to the ward. I said that I was pregnant. I did the test and was shown the negative result. I was given Risperdal that made me feel much better.

"That's what I need! Risperdal will help me!" I thought. I did not stay in the hospital - they let me go home. I could no longer stay at home and decided to take Chavi to the neighbors.

I tied him with a long leash and left him there. "Where I am going?", I thought. I saw some Indians open the balcony door on the first floor. I walked over and greeted them. I asked if I could come in. The old couple agreed. I told them that my boyfriend was beating me. I watched Edward my dog-lover friend to bring Chavi food and water. Then the house manager came to take Chavi.

I spent a few hours with the Indians and then their son came over. He tried to send me away, but I said I did not want to go. Soon the police arrived and led me outside. The police car took me to Saint Mary. After sitting in the queue, I was led into the room. I said that I was pregnant. I did a test and was said I was not, they gave me a pill and soon I was discharged.

Once I got home, I told Yigal that the house manager took Chavi. In the morning, I attacked her. I told her to give my dog back or I would call the police. Yigal returned from work and said that the house manager had taken Chavi to the pound. We went there and took Chavi home.

The house manager said if we did not stop piddling around, we would be evicted. I stopped calling the fire brigade and police.

One day Yigal and I went to the cinema to watch "Beowulf" with Angelina Jolie. When I got home later on, I heard the voice of a woman.

"She scattered her gold!" I remember when I was in the hospital I threw away the golden chain - Yigal's gift. "Go back to Israel, stop stealing our fiancés!"

There was a thunderstorm in the evening. I came up to the window to look at the storm.

Suddenly the voice of God ordered "Geula go away!" But I had not moved. Suddenly the lightning struck the road near our house. I jumped into bed stunned. Yigal was sleeping and in the morning took me to the Saint Mary then I ended up in the psychiatric ward.

I saw the doctor at Saint Mary Hospital. I laughingly told him that I should not do ECT. The storm has already done everything. I asked for Risperdal.

"I'll give you Risperdal" - the doctor said while standing up.

I had my lunch in the canteen when I saw a man with a large suitcase coming out of the hospital doors.

I was talking to a patient. I asked him if he believed in demons. He said they were existing somewhere in our lives.

"I can hear them", I replied.

They took a blood test and prescribed me six milligrams of Risperdal. Three days later, I was discharged. I was getting better; the child's voice had gone. I was not in a psychotic state. Six milligrams of Risperdal helped me.

Psychotic state was over. But I kept hearing the voices of demons.

One day I heard a woman's voice. "You are bewitched. Go to the Christians" she said.

"The Christians should not be here! Chavi is ours. She does not like our stuff", said the demon. "They've got a truck. They put someone in a truck and take to the Devil", the woman said. I did not know how to get rid of these voices.

I offered Yigal to swap our rooms so he would hear the voices. He could not hear anything. I thought they remained silent because Yigal was in my room.

After some time, many bills came in the mail of more than $25,000. This was the sum of all the ambulances and fire department services, hospitalizations and medications. Fortunately, Medicaid paid the bills.

Wayne Dyer

Yigal was experiencing the events caused by my illness and tried to find remedies to my situation. He tried to find in places that are outside the realm of the medical world.

One day we watched a PBS show on television where Dr. Wayne Dyer spoke about: the need to fulfill your dharma and find a way to change circumstances. He was talking about what happens when you do what you really want to do in your life. When you do that, he said, the entire universe would help you to fulfill it. He talked about synchronicity – where you collaborate with fate. Suddenly the right people show up in your life the right events and things like money resources and possibilities arrive to you. He also said that in order to get this done you must practice imagining or exercising your brain to the state where your aim is already being fulfilled.

I wanted to make high quality dolls, make jewelry, and to build and promote websites on the internet. Yigal told me please give it a try.

Every day Yigal and me imagined me getting better and I started to build a greeting cards website I always wanted to build. Then a sequence of events took place that would eventually substantially diminish my illness.

In Canada

Yigal got laid off from his job and we moved to Canada. We rented a house in Toronto. We had a haunted spirit at home.

He used to say "The bread is delicious" when I left him a hunk of bread at night.

"I am hungry" he said and I left the fruits on the table. Yigal did not hear him but I did. The voices of demons chased me even here.

"Walking organs" they called me. The doctors said that brain tricks me that it is only in my mind. But excuse me, I would never call a person "Walking organs". Only someone very evilminded can say that.

I decided to go to Church and talk to the Pastor. I came to the Pastor and told him that demons haunted me. She offered to bless my house. But I said that it was not in the house but inside of me. Wherever I lived demons were haunted me. She gave me the phone number of the social worker. I called the social worker and made an appointment. I told my story in the meeting. She said I need a doctor. But this was not new to me.

Back to Israel

Yigal and I returned to Israel. I went to a private doctor Bella Grinwitch. She wasn't a conventional doctor in the sense that she did not administer her patients only one drug but a "cocktail" of them.

It took several weeks but eventually we found my suitable combination. In the morning I take: 8mg Perphinan 5mg Zyprexa and 10mg Vaben. At noon I take: 3mg of Risperdal, 5mg Zyprexa and 10mg Vaben. In the evening: 8mg Perphinan and 3mg Risperdal. Also I take from time to time when I cannot sleep Brotizolam. Because of Perphinan Demonic voices disappeared. This keeps me in almost a perfect health free from hallucinations and enables me to function as a normal person.

I live quietly since then. No more psychotic attacks and of course with Yigal's infinite love. But I had never known whether Mal was Satan or a prince. Yigal is my real prince.

Sanity

This book documents the psychotic condition I was in. Here I would like to tell you what is behind the story; medical wise as well how to maintain good quality of life.

The trigger for the first stroke was pressure at work, the second was due to stopping the administration of Iloperidone and the third was due to taking acne prevention supplements. Any change in dosage may trigger psychotic behavior.

From the sequence of events depicted here one can understand that an unbalanced schizophrenia patient's quality of life does not enable him to function normally in life and he must be watched all the time by someone healthy. Many actions prohibit him from keeping the very basic functions of life. Actions like: working at a regular job to earn living, communicating with the surroundings, distinguishing between imagination and reality, buying groceries, going to the cinema (i.e. due to high volume of sound), to go out to restaurants in crowded places, take care of personal hygiene and also studying.

I would distinguish between two levels of schizophrenic behavior: a full psychotic condition where voice and visional hallucinations occur where the patient has to be hospitalized, and "semi-balanced" condition where the patient has voices hallucinations seldom occurring– the patient is at home.

In the case of full psychotic event the patient has to know what is real and imaginary. This is done by conversing with the healthy person prior to the event and building an absolute, trusting relationship.

This means that when the event occurs the healthy person can ask the patient: "Have I ever lied to you?", name the hallucinations and identifying them: what is real and what is not. The patient thus is in a psychotic situation but the fact that there is a distinction between false and true reality will calm him a bit and thus lower the strength of psychotic condition.

Also the healthy person should try to fulfill every wish of the patient because this keeps the validation of the truthfulness of the relation with the healthy person and calms the patient. This does not mean that the need for medication can be eliminated in the case of psychotic behavior, but it put some control over it. Anyway hospitalization is necessary.

In the case of the patient living at home there are reasons for the change in condition digressing from perfect health. These are forms of pressure present in life. The healthy person overlooking the patient has to identify this digression and talk to the patient identifying the cause and try to actively create different circumstances. In my case for example, if I work more than four hours a day then after several days I develop voice hallucinations.

I hope that this book describes well a story of a Schizophrenia patient. I would also like give hope to patients and doctors that the life of schizophrenia patients can be improved.

www.ingramcontent.com/pod-product-compliance
Lightning Source LLC
Chambersburg PA
CBHW051707170526
45167CB00002B/569